Introduction

Early Intervention Developmental Profile is a compilation of major developmental milestones for use with children whose cognitive, motor, social, self-care, and/or language skills fall within the 0 to 36-month developmental range. The profile provides a systematic means of evaluating a child's skills, selecting appropriate objectives for treatment of developmental delays, and designing an appropriate, individualized curriculum based on a developmental model.

The profile evaluates the child's functioning in six areas: perceptual/fine motor, cognition, language, social/emotional, self-care, and gross motor. The profile is designed to be administered up to four times a year for one child by an interdisciplinary team which includes a psychologist or special educator, physical and/or occupational therapist, and a speech therapist. Each section of the profile assumes a certain degree of disciplinary knowledge and skill on the part of the evaluator, skills which can be taught to other members of the team.

Scoring procedures for each item are described in volume 1, *Assessment and Application,* of the five-volume set *Developmental Programming for Infants and Young Children.* Briefly, an item *passed* by the child is marked with a P if the criteria are met. When there is a question as to whether the child has fully met the criteria for an item, a *pass-fail* (PF) should be used to indicate the emergence of the skill measured by that particular item. Clear *failures* are marked by an F. A final scoring category, O, is used to signify that an item has been *omitted* by the evaluator because of intervening variables which should be described in the scoring box.

The child's performance can be plotted on the profile graph (inside back cover) by marking the highest item number of a sequence of passes the child earned in each of the six areas and then connecting the marks. The resulting graph provides a visual representation of the child's relative strengths, weaknesses, and general developmental level. Objectives for the child in each developmental area can be designed to aid the acquisition of skills in the appropriate developmental level, supporting the strong (highest) skills as well as facilitating the development of the weak (lowest) area(s). The process of translating evaluation data into individualized programs is fully discussed in volume 1.

The materials necessary to administer the entire profile are listed below:

Flashlight
Rattle
Bell
Small doll
Bottle for doll
Dish
Mirror
Balls, small (4-inch diameter)
    medium (8-inch diameter)
Paper-wrapped candy
Toy car
Toys that represent household items
Cloth or diaper
Sponge

Baby bottle
Three identical coffee cups
Small jar and lid (not more than 2
    inches in diameter)
Card with pictures of girl and boy
Three-piece body puzzle
12-inch stick
Small square box
Two sets of cards with four geometric
    shapes—circle, square, star, cross
Penny
Ring on string
Raisins or sugar pellets
Six pegs (3/8-inch to 1/2-inch diameter)

Six-holed pegboard
5 crayons
Paper
Picture book with cardboard pages
Three-piece formboard
Blunt-end scissors
Pull toy
Stairs
Eight 1/2-inch beads with two strings
5 spoons
Six red cards/six yellow cards
Ten 1-inch cubes—two each of red, blue, yellow, green, black
1/2-inch cube

Small clear vial
Food and utensils (including fork)
Drinking straw
Comb or hairbrush
Washcloth
Zipper
Child-sized chair
Adult-sized chair
Balance beam
Tricycle
Small toys which can fit under inverted coffee cups
Sample sheet pictures

ITEM NUMBER	DEVELOPMENTAL LEVELS AND ITEMS	DATE	DATE	DATE	DATE
	0–2 months				
*1	Responds to different light intensities				
2	Focuses momentarily on face or soft light				
3	Follows moving object horizontally and vertically				
4	Follows moving object through most of a circular path				
	3–5 months				
*5	Integration of grasp reflex				
6	Reaches for dangling object				
7	Moves head to track moving object				
8	Fingers own hands in play at midline				
9	Uses ulnar palmar prehension				
10	Reaches for cube and touches it				
11	Uses radial palmar prehension (uses thumb and two fingers)				
12	Transfers toy from hand to hand				
	6–8 months				
13	Pulls one peg out of pegboard				
14	Rakes or scoops up raisin and attains it				
15	Has complete thumb opposition on cube				
16	Uses inferior pincer grasp with raisin				
	9–11 months				
17	Pokes with isolated index finger				
18	Drops a block with voluntary release				
19	Uses neat pincer grasp with raisin				
20	Attempts to imitate scribble (holds crayon to paper)				
21	Holds crayon adaptively				

* = reflex, righting reaction, protective response, or equilibrium reaction

Developmental Programming for Infants and Young Children
Volume 2: Early Intervention Developmental Profile

Perceptual/Fine Motor

ITEM NUMBER	DEVELOPMENTAL LEVELS AND ITEMS	DATE	DATE	DATE	DATE

12–15 months

ITEM NUMBER	DEVELOPMENTAL LEVELS AND ITEMS	DATE	DATE	DATE	DATE
22	Turns page of cardboard book				
23	Removes cover from small square box				
24	Places one or two pegs in pegboard				
25	Builds two-cube tower				
26	Scribbles spontaneously (no demonstration)				
27	Releases raisin into small bottle				

16–19 months

ITEM NUMBER	DEVELOPMENTAL LEVELS AND ITEMS	DATE	DATE	DATE	DATE
28	Places six pegs in pegboard without help				
29	Builds three-cube tower				
30	Places round form in formboard (three forms presented)				
31	Imitates crayon stroke				

20–23 months

ITEM NUMBER	DEVELOPMENTAL LEVELS AND ITEMS	DATE	DATE	DATE	DATE
32	Places six pegs in pegboard in 34 seconds				
33	Makes vertical and circular scribble after demonstration				
34	Completes three-piece formboard				
35	Builds six-cube tower				
36	Holds crayon with fingers				
37	Attempts to fold paper imitatively				

24–27 months

ITEM NUMBER	DEVELOPMENTAL LEVELS AND ITEMS	DATE	DATE	DATE	DATE
38	Draws vertical and horizontal strokes imitatively				
39	Completes reversed formboard				
40	Aligns two or more cubes for train, no smokestack				
41	Unscrews jar lid				
42	Scribbles with circular motion				

ITEM NUMBER	*DEVELOPMENTAL LEVELS AND ITEMS*	DATE	DATE	DATE	DATE
	28–31 months				
43	Builds eight-cube tower				
44	Aligns three cubes for train with smokestack				
45	Imitates paper folding				
	32–35 months				
46	Copies a circle already drawn				
47	Cuts with scissors				
48	Strings five ½-inch beads				

Developmental Programming for Infants and Young Children
Volume 2: Early Intervention Developmental Profile

ITEM NUMBER	*DEVELOPMENTAL LEVELS AND ITEMS*	DATE	DATE	DATE	DATE
	0–2 months				
49	Uses adaptive movements rather than reflexive reactions				
50	Brings hand to mouth				
51	Repeats random movements				
	3–5 months				
52	Mouths object				
53	Shakes rattle				
54	Looks at object s/he is holding				
55	Tracks rolling ball momentarily screened				
	6–8 months				
56	Attains partially hidden object				
57	Looks to the floor when something falls				
58	Uncovers face				
59	Bangs object				
60	Rotates a bottle inverted less than 180° to drink				
61	Imitates hand movements already in his/her repertoire				
	9–11 months				
62	Attains completely hidden object				
63	Pulls string to secure ring and succeeds				
64	Shows knowledge of toy hidden behind a screen				
65	Imitates facial movements inexactly				
66	Imperfectly imitates movements never performed before				
67	Rotates a bottle inverted 180° to drink				
68	Reacts to novel features of an object				

ITEM NUMBER	*DEVELOPMENTAL LEVELS AND ITEMS*	DATE	DATE	DATE	DATE
	12–15 months				
69	Imitates body action on a doll				
70	Repeatedly finds toy when hidden under one of several covers				
71	Lifts a ½-inch cube off a 1-inch cube				
72	Balances nine 1-inch cubes in a coffee cup				
	16–19 months				
73	Repeatedly finds toy when hidden under multiple covers				
74	Uses a stick to try to attain an object out of reach				
75	Retrieves raisin by inverting small vial				
76	Corrects imitations of new movements				
77	Deduces location of hidden object, single displacement				
78	Pulls cloth to reach object				
	20–23 months				
79	Imitates unseen body movements immediately and exactly				
80	Attempts to activate flashlight				
81	Deduces location of hidden object, multiple displacements				
82	Anticipates path of rolling ball by detouring around object				
83	Matches two sets of objects by item				
	24–27 months				
84	Imitates a model from memory				
85	Matches two sets of objects by color				
86	Assembles three-piece body puzzle correctly				
87	Recognizes four pictures from reduced cues				

Cognition

ITEM NUMBER	DEVELOPMENTAL LEVELS AND ITEMS	DATE	DATE	DATE	DATE
	28–31 months				
88	Matches colored cubes (red, yellow, blue, green, black)				
89	Understands concept of one				
90	Identifies three objects by their use (car, penny, bottle)				
	32–35 months				
91	Repeats two digits				
92	Matches four shapes (circle, square, star, cross)				
93	Inverts a picture				
94	Names a missing object				

ITEM NUMBER	*DEVELOPMENTAL LEVELS AND ITEMS*	DATE	DATE	DATE	DATE

Notation in parentheses following each test item indicates that the response is either receptive language (R), expressive language (E), or imitative behavior (I).

0–2 months

95	Moves limbs, head, eyes in response to voice, noise (R)				
96	Vocalizes randomly (E)				

3–5 months

97	Vocalizes when talked to or sung to (E)				
98	Turns eyes or head in direction of voices and sounds (R)				
99	Exhibits differentiated crying (E)				
100	Vocalizes emotions, intonation patterns (E)				

6–8 months

101	Vocalizes consonant sounds (E)				
102	Localizes sound source (R)				
103	Forms bisyllabic repetitions (ma-ma, ba-ba)(E)				
104	Imitates sounds already in repertoire (I)				

9–11 months

105	Orients to spoken name (R)				
106	Imitates consonant-vowel combinations (I)				
107	Performs on verbal cue alone (R)				
108	Imitates nonspeech sounds (click, cough)(I)				
109	Inhibits activity in response to **no** (R)				
110	Looks at familiar objects or persons when named (R)				

12–15 months

111	Uses appropriate intonation patterns in jargon speech (E)				

Developmental Programming for Infants and Young Children
Volume 2: Early Intervention Developmental Profile

ITEM NUMBER	DEVELOPMENTAL LEVELS AND ITEMS	DATE	DATE	DATE	DATE
112	Imitates words inexactly (I)				
113	Uses two words meaningfully (E)				
114	Uses gestures and other movements to communicate (E)				
115	Follows a simple direction (R)				
116	Shows a body part, clothing item, or toy on verbal request (R)				

16–19 months

ITEM NUMBER	DEVELOPMENTAL LEVELS AND ITEMS	DATE	DATE	DATE	DATE
117	Names one object on request (E)				
118	Follows two familiar directions (R)				
119	Points to one black and white picture on request (R)				
120	Uses more than two single words to express wants (E)				
121	Points to three body parts on self or doll (R)				
122	Names one black and white picture (E)				
123	Selects two of three familiar objects (R)				

20–23 months

ITEM NUMBER	DEVELOPMENTAL LEVELS AND ITEMS	DATE	DATE	DATE	DATE
124	Points to four pictures (R)				
125	Uses two-word sentences (E)				
126	Names at least three familiar objects or pictures (E)				
127	Imitates new sounds and simple words immediately (I)				
128	Follows a new instruction exactly (R)				

24–27 months

ITEM NUMBER	DEVELOPMENTAL LEVELS AND ITEMS	DATE	DATE	DATE	DATE
129	Uses own name when referring to self (E)				
130	Uses three-word sentences (E)				
131	Uses four different semantic functions (E)				

28–31 months

ITEM NUMBER	DEVELOPMENTAL LEVELS AND ITEMS	DATE	DATE	DATE	DATE
132	Responds appropriately to two requests regarding location (R)				

ITEM NUMBER	DEVELOPMENTAL LEVELS AND ITEMS	DATE	DATE	DATE	DATE
133	Uses three different sentence types (E)				
134	Answers questions regarding body part functions (E)				

32–35 months

ITEM NUMBER	DEVELOPMENTAL LEVELS AND ITEMS	DATE	DATE	DATE	DATE
135	Uses four different grammatic constructions appropriately (E)				

ITEM NUMBER	*DEVELOPMENTAL LEVELS AND ITEMS*	DATE	DATE	DATE	DATE
0–2 months					
136	Quiets when picked up				
137	Quiets to face or voice				
138	Maintains brief periods of eye contact during feeding				
139	Smiles or vocalizes to talk and touch				
3–5 months					
140	Watches adult walk across room				
141	Reflects silent adult's smile				
142	Smiles or reaches to familiar people				
143	Smiles or laughs during physical play				
144	Smiles spontaneously				
145	Smiles at image in mirror				
6–8 months					
146	Prefers to be with people				
147	Laughs and smiles at pat-a-cake and peek-a-boo games				
148	Reaches for image of self in mirror				
149	Explores features of a familiar person				
9–11 months					
150	Leaves physical contact with familiar person momentarily				
151	Participates in pat-a-cake and peek-a-boo games				
152	Performs for social attention				
153	Offers toy				
12–15 months					
154	Responds differentially to young children				
155	Gives toy to adult				

ITEM NUMBER	DEVELOPMENTAL LEVELS AND ITEMS	DATE	DATE	DATE	DATE
156	Initiates ball play or social games				
157	Leaves contact with familiar person repeatedly				

16–19 months

ITEM NUMBER	DEVELOPMENTAL LEVELS AND ITEMS	DATE	DATE	DATE	DATE
158	Plays apart from familiar person for 5 minutes				
159	Varies play with one toy				
160	Approaches a young child				

20–23 months

ITEM NUMBER	DEVELOPMENTAL LEVELS AND ITEMS	DATE	DATE	DATE	DATE
161	Occasionally plays near other children				
162	Shows periods of strong independence				
163	Picks up and puts away toys on request				
164	Imitates domestic activities				

24–27 months

ITEM NUMBER	DEVELOPMENTAL LEVELS AND ITEMS	DATE	DATE	DATE	DATE
165	Independently chooses toy and begins to play				
166	Pretends to be engaged in familiar activities (being asleep, telephoning)				
167	Prefers to play near, but not with, other children				

28–31 months

ITEM NUMBER	DEVELOPMENTAL LEVELS AND ITEMS	DATE	DATE	DATE	DATE
168	Discriminates between boys and girls				
169	Identifies self in mirror				
170	Plays with other children				

32–35 months

ITEM NUMBER	DEVELOPMENTAL LEVELS AND ITEMS	DATE	DATE	DATE	DATE
171	Separates from familiar person in strange environment for 5 minutes				
172	Identifies own sex				
173	Shares toy with adult prompts				

Developmental Programming for Infants and Young Children
Volume 2: Early Intervention Developmental Profile

ITEM NUMBER	DEVELOPMENTAL LEVELS AND ITEMS	DATE	DATE	DATE	DATE
Feeding Skills	**0–2 months**				
*174	Sucks well from bottle or breast				
175	Coordinates sucking, swallowing, and breathing				
	3–5 months				
176	Sucks and swallows pureed foods from spoon				
*177	Integration of rooting reflex				
178	Gums or mouths pureed food				
*179	Integration of bite reflex				
	6–8 months				
180	Gums and swallows cracker				
181	Closes lips on spoon to remove food				
182	Drinks from cup with help				
183	Picks up spoon				
184	Chews with lateral tongue motion				
	9–11 months				
185	Finger feeds small pieces of food				
186	Bites cracker				
187	Chews cracker				
188	Licks food off spoon				
189	Eats mashed table foods				
190	Ceases drooling				
191	Swallows with closed mouth				
	12–15 months				
192	Feeds self with spoon (many spills)				
193	Picks up and drinks from cup (some spilling)				
194	Chews well				

ITEM NUMBER	DEVELOPMENTAL LEVELS AND ITEMS	DATE	DATE	DATE	DATE
	16–19 months				
195	Drinks from cup without assistance				
196	Eats with spoon independently (entire meal)				
197	Discriminates edibles				
	20–23 months				
198	Unwraps candy; peels or pits fruit				
199	Sucks through a straw				
	24–35 months				
200	Begins to use fork				
201	Gets drink without help				
202	Spoon feeds (no spilling)				
Toileting Skills	**12–15 months**				
203	Remains dry for 1 to 2 hour periods				
204	Fusses to be changed				
	16–23 months				
205	Has regular bowel movements				
206	Begins toilet training				
	24–35 months				
207	Remains dry between regular toileting				
208	Uses gestures or words to indicate need to use toilet				
209	Toilets independently except for wiping				
210	Has infrequent bowel accidents				
Dressing/Hygiene Skills	**12–15 months**				
211	Pulls off hat, socks, or mittens on request				
212	Cooperates in diapering and dressing by moving limbs				

Developmental Programming for Infants and Young Children
Volume 2: Early Intervention Developmental Profile

ITEM NUMBER	DEVELOPMENTAL LEVELS AND ITEMS	DATE	DATE	DATE	DATE
213	Attempts to brush hair				

16–19 months

ITEM NUMBER	DEVELOPMENTAL LEVELS AND ITEMS	DATE	DATE	DATE	DATE
214	Attempts to wash face or hands				
215	Cooperates with toothbrushing				

20–23 months

ITEM NUMBER	DEVELOPMENTAL LEVELS AND ITEMS	DATE	DATE	DATE	DATE
216	Undresses completely except for fastenings				
217	Attempts to put shoes on				
218	Unzips and zips large zipper				

24–31 months

ITEM NUMBER	DEVELOPMENTAL LEVELS AND ITEMS	DATE	DATE	DATE	DATE
219	Puts on simple clothes without assistance (e.g., hat, pants, shoes)				
220	Washes and dries hands with assistance				

32–35 months

ITEM NUMBER	DEVELOPMENTAL LEVELS AND ITEMS	DATE	DATE	DATE	DATE
221	Dries hands independently				
222	Puts on coat, dress, T-shirt except for buttoning				
223	Undoes large buttons, snaps, shoelaces deliberately				

ITEM NUMBER	DEVELOPMENTAL LEVELS AND ITEMS	DATE	DATE	DATE	DATE
	0–2 months				
224	Prone: turns head to both sides				
*225	Neck righting				
226	Upright: head bobs but stays erect				
*227	Prone: optical righting				
228	Prone: raises and maintains head at 45°				
229	Supine: kicks feet alternately				
	3–5 months				
*230	Integration of Moro reflex				
231	Prone: head and chest are raised to 90° with forearm support				
232	Upright: bears small fraction of weight on feet				
233	Prone: props with extended arms				
234	Aligns head with trunk when pulled to sitting				
235	Pulls self to sitting				
236	Prone: rolls to supine				
*237	Prone: integration of tonic labyrinthine reflex (TLR)				
*238	Supine: integration of tonic labyrinthine reflex (TLR)				
*239	Prone: integration of symmetrical tonic neck reflex (STNR)				
*240	Supine: integration of asymmetrical tonic neck reflex (ATNR)				
	6–8 months				
241	Sitting: trunk erect in chair				
242	Upright: extends legs and takes large fraction of weight				
243	Prone: reaches				
244	Prone: assumes quadruped				

ITEM NUMBER	DEVELOPMENTAL LEVELS AND ITEMS	DATE	DATE	DATE	DATE
*245	Body on body righting begins				
246	Sits unsupported for 30 seconds				
*247	Supine: optical righting				
*248	Prone: Landau response				
*249	Sitting: protective extension to the front				
*250	Parachute reaction				
*251	Sitting: optical righting when tipped to sides				
252	Supine: rolls to prone				
253	Prone: pivots				
254	Prone: crawls				
*255	Sitting: protective extension to the sides				
256	Standing: moves body up and down				
257	Sitting: assists in pulling to standing				
258	Supine: rotates to sitting and quadruped				

9–11 months

ITEM NUMBER	DEVELOPMENTAL LEVELS AND ITEMS	DATE	DATE	DATE	DATE
259	Standing: takes one step when supported				
260	Quadruped: creeps				
*261	Sitting: protective extension to the rear				
262	Sitting: pulls to standing using furniture				
263	Standing: lowers self to floor				
264	Standing: cruises by holding on to furniture				
265	Walks with one hand held				
*266	Sitting: equilibrium reactions				
267	Stands alone				
*268	Quadruped: equilibrium reactions				

12–15 months

ITEM NUMBER	DEVELOPMENTAL LEVELS AND ITEMS	DATE	DATE	DATE	DATE
269	Walks by him/herself				
270	Creeps up stairs				

ITEM NUMBER	DEVELOPMENTAL LEVELS AND ITEMS	DATE	DATE	DATE	DATE
271	Standing: throws ball with some cast				
272	Walks well (stops, starts, turns)				
273	Supine: raises self to standing position independently				
274	Walks backward				
275	Squats in play, resumes standing position				

16–19 months

276	"Runs" stiffly				
277	Walks sideways				
278	Walks up stairs held by one hand				
279	Creeps backward down stairs				
280	Standing: seats self in small chair				
281	Climbs into adult-sized chair				
282	Standing: balances on one foot with help				
*283	Standing: equilibrium reactions				

20–23 months

284	Walks down stairs with one hand held				
285	Jumps in place				

24–27 months

286	Goes up and down stairs alone, nonreciprocally				
287	Stands on balance beam with both feet; attempts to step				
288	Kicks ball				
289	Jumps from bottom step (feet together)				

28–31 months

290	Walks on tiptoes				
291	Throws ball 5 to 7 feet in a vertical pattern				
292	Takes a few alternate steps on balance beam				
293	Supine: rises to standing with mature pattern				

ITEM NUMBER	DEVELOPMENTAL LEVELS AND ITEMS	DATE	DATE	DATE	DATE
	32–35 months				
294	Rides tricycle using pedals				
295	Goes up stairs alternating feet				
296	Stands on one foot and balances				
297	Walks with heel-toe gait				
298	Walks with reciprocal arm swing				
299	Runs				

Developmental Programming for Infants and Young Children
Volume 2: Early Intervention Developmental Profile

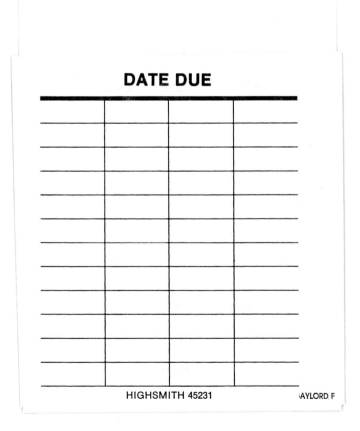

DATE DUE

HIGHSMITH 45231   AYLORD F